Ayurveda
A beginner's guide to natural health and well-being for every aspect of your life

SARAH R. GRAY

Image use under CC-BY License via Flickrr

Spices. Photo credit: Sammy JayJay

ISBN: 1503351017

ISBN-13: 978-1503351011

When diet is wrong medicine is of no use.
When diet is correct medicine is of no need.
~Ayurvedic Proverb.

CONTENTS

1 INTRODUCTION TO AYURVEDA

Why is alternative medicine becoming more popular and mainstream? Because it's simply effective and is free from synthetic chemicals that can cause adverse effects to your overall well-being. From reducing the side-effects of chemotherapy to treating psychiatric disorders like depression and anxiety, alternative medicine has the uncanny ability to treat a wide variety of maladies in a very safe and efficient fashion. Not to mention, alternative therapies are far cheaper than surgical treatments.

Ayurveda: A powerful form of alternative medicine

When it comes to holistic health and natural therapies, Ayurveda may not be the first thing that comes into your mind. When people talk about natural treatments and therapies, they will normally mention yoga, acupuncture and massage. While this ancient practice is not as popular as its contemporaries, it is nonetheless a powerful system that can greatly benefit your health in a lot of different ways.

What is Ayurveda? Also, how can it help me with my medical conditions? Well, Ayurveda, or also referred as Ayurvedic medicine, is an ancient Hindu practice that maintains your health by keeping your spirit, mind and body in perfect serenity with nature. Developed over two thousand years ago in India, this one-of-a-kind alternative therapy is truly one of the oldest holistic natural healing systems in the world. As a traditional holistic system, Ayurveda mainly focuses on promoting good health, instead of fighting conditions and diseases. But, there are treatments that can be arranged for specific conditions and health problems. Of course, these treatments are handled by licensed Ayurvedic practitioners.

"We can't talk about our own health without understanding our place in our environment, because in order to fulfill our potential we have to live in the content of our surroundings. We have to known our place in the ecosystem of which we are a part, and this means living consciously: being aware of nature and how it affects us and how we, in turn, affect nature."

- Sebastian Pole, Discovering the True You with Ayurveda

Ayurveda, though, is more than just a system for preventing and treating conditions. Derived from the Sanskrit words, ayur (life) and veda (knowledge), Ayurveda is practically a body of knowledge designed to aid people in staying vital, as they try to reach their full potential as human beings. What's more, this ancient practice provides insightful guidelines on your ideal seasonal and daily routines, behavior, diet as well as the proper use of your senses. Indeed, it is holistic approach that can make you a better, healthier and more knowledgeable person.

Deepak Chopra, a prominent advocate of alternative medicine, is the man many considered responsible for introducing Ayurveda to the modern pop culture. As a believer and practitioner of Ayurveda, Dr. Chopra has shared the concepts of this holistic system to other distinguished media figures like Oprah and Lady Gaga. Likewise, he has witnessed all the healing properties of this compelling holistic art.

"By balance, I mean a return to what in medical terms or biological terms is called homeostasis, self-regulation. So any disease, doesn't matter what it is, is a disruption in homeostasis. And in the integrated approach of Ayurveda, and many other traditional healing systems, all you're doing is using different modalities to restore the original state of balance. Ayurveda is useful in any chronic illness. Coronary artery disease, rheumatoid arthritis or other inflammations. Bronchial asthma, obesity, type 2 diabetes. Because these are all linked to lifestyle".

-   Deepak Chopra M.D.

In addition to Dr. Chopra, there have been an awful lot of other famous personalities that trust and believe in Ayurvedic medicine. Christy Turlington, a sensational and highly acclaimed supermodel, is one of the numerous celebrities to have enjoyed the perks of this compelling medical system. As an Ayurvedic practitioner, Christy believes that Ayurveda that improves health, mind and beauty.

Origins

As with other ancient practices, Ayurveda has a very rich and colorful history. Shared originally as a Hindu oral tradition, Ayurvedic medicine was first recorded over five thousand years ago in Sanskrit. As historians have said, this ancient practice was recorded in Vedas, a tetrad of sacred texts that include Atharva Veda (1200-1000 BCE), Sam Veda, Yajur Veda and Rig Veda (3000-2500 BCE). By the way, the Vedas books state the knowledge of Ayurvedic medicine was given directly by Brahma, who Ayurveda practitioners believe is the architect of the world.

Books in Ayurvedic medicine become available in the 8th century BCE. As medical books, these texts not only feature procedural instructions, but it also contains history lessons on how this medical system has evolved through time.

There are three early primary texts about this holistic system, all dating back to the Common Era's earlier centuries. These early texts are the

Sushruta Samhita, Chakara Samhita, as well as the medical parts of Bheda Samhita (Bower Manuscript). Of the three texts, the Chakara Samhita is considered the ultimate source. The original Chakara Samhita was made around 100 BCE to 100 CE, while the Sushruta Samhita was written either in the third or fourth century. Bheda Samhita, meanwhile, was written in the earlier parts of the 6th century.

In 1500 BC, Ayurveda was divided into eight branches, namely:

Internal Medicine (Kaaya Chikitsa)

Pediatrics (Baala Chikitsa)

Psychology or Demonology (Graha Chikitsa)

Treatment of ailments that are above the human clavicle (Urdhvaanga Chikitsa)

Surgery (Shalya Chikitsa)

Toxicology (Damstra Chikitsa)

Rejuvenation or Geriatrics (Jara Chikitsa)

Aphrodisiac therapy (Vrsha Chikitsa)

Also, in that span of time, there were a couple of main schools designed for Ayurvedic medicine, the Dhanvantari (school of surgeons) and Atria (school of physicians). With the advent of these two schools, Ayurveda became a more scientifically classifiable and verifiable medical system.

In modern times, Ayurveda has flourished into a highly respected medical system in India. In fact, this ancient practice is now well integrated into the national healthcare system of India, with a handful of Ayurvedic hospitals established all over the country. Moreover, hordes of medical practitioners from all over the world flock to Ayurvedic schools in India, to learn this age-old holistic approach.

With the numerous holistic benefits that can be offered by Ayurveda, it is no wonder millions of people from all corners of the world are now getting Ayurvedic treatments. From sports injuries, spinal disorders and chronic pain to respiratory problems, this ancient Indian practice has been widely used in curing a broad range of maladies and conditions. Plus, it is a potent beauty care solution that helps prevent aging, hair loss and weight gain. So, if you want to be as healthy as Dr. Chopra, and look as stunning as Christy Turlington, consider becoming a follower of this flourishing health trend.

2 THE THREE DOSHAS OF AYURVEDA

Have you ever asked yourself why people are very different from one another? Why do some people exude stillness and grace, while others are fast-moving with boundless energy? Why can some barely finish a sandwich, while others can easily finish a 5-course meal? Why do others feel like their carrying the weight of the world, while some are just naturally joyous?

In spite of recent developments in the world of science of medicine, experts cannot find concrete answers to some of the questions stated above. Sure, modern genetics provide some helpful insights, but it doesn't have solid data pertaining to the idiosyncrasies and characteristics that make each person unique. Thankfully, Ayurveda can shed some light on these mysteries, with its three doshas, Kapha, Pitta and Vata.

"Anyone who believes that anything can be suited to everyone is a great fool, because medicine is practiced not on mankind on general, but on every individual in particular."

-   Henri de Mondeville

About the doshas

In Ayurvedic medicine, doshas are referred to the biological energies that are found throughout the mind and body. As your biological energy, your dosha governs all your mental and physical processes as well as provide you with a distinctive blueprint for fulfillment and health.

These fundamental energies are derived from the world's five elements, and the properties related to them. Vata, for instance, has the qualities that reflect the elements of air and space. Pitta, on other hand, has qualities that bespeak the elements of water and fire. As for Kapha, it is a fundamental energy with qualities that reflect the elements of earth and water. For every element, there is an imbalanced and balanced expression. To get a deeper and better understanding about these energies and elements, take a look at the description of each dosha type below.

Vata people

An individual, who is predominantly Vata, will have mental and physical qualities that exhibit the elemental qualities of air and space. For that reason, Vata people are usually hyperactive and fast-thinkers. Just like a wind that provides expression and movement to the world, a well-balanced Vata person is also creative, active, and naturally gifted with the ability to communicate and express his or her thoughts. But when his or her wind rages like a storm, the person's negative qualities will instantly overshadow his or her positive traits and attributes. The most prevalent signs of a Vata person having an imbalance include dryness (like constipation and dry skin), bodily disorders and anxiety.

Vata qualities: changeable, quick, moving, rough, irregular, dry, light and cold

Of the three doshas, Vata stands atop as the most important one. Not only does it directly influence the other two doshas, but it is also your body's main mover or driver, controlling your waste products and tissues.

Functions of Vata

> Controls all eliminations, such as sweat, urine, feces, semen and fetus.

> Aids in metabolism.

> Controls a variety of mental and physical movements in the body, from muscle contraction to respiration.

> Relays all the sensory inputs from various sense organs to your brain.

Pitta People

As a dosha derived from the elements of water and fire, Pitta people will display mental and physical characteristics that reflect the qualities of these two elements. When a Pitta person is in perfect balance, he or she will have a joyful vibe or disposition. Not to mention, a balanced Pitta individual will have tremendous drive and courage as well as a rather sharp intellect. But when the fire of the person's body and mind becomes rowdy, a blissful Pitta oddly transforms into screeching one. As ego, rage and anger overcome his or her positive traits, the imbalanced Pitta becomes a bitter person with no positive outlook in life. As Ayurvedic practitioners say, imbalanced Pittas won't go to hell, as they would practically make it everywhere they go.

Pitta qualities: acidic, liquid, moving, light, hot, sharp and oily

Functions of Pitta

Aids in metabolisms at all levels, from food digestion to transformation.

Helps maintain the ideal body temperature.

Transforms external images into impulses of your optic nerves.

Controls appetite.

Gives softness and color to your skin.

Braveness and courage.

Comprehension.

Kapha People

Reflecting the elements of water and earth, a Kapha person will normally have a calm temperament and compact body frame. When a Kapha is in good balance, he or she will display positive qualities, such as being stable, supportive and sweet. But when he or she is out of balance, the Kapha individual may experience congestion, sinus, weight gain and sluggishness.

Kapha qualities: Oily, soft, cold, solid, steady, slow, heavy

Functions of Kapha

> Virility and fertility.
>
> Structure and mass.
>
> Stability.
>
> Helps prevent excessive friction from happening between several parts of your body.
>
> Aids in performing physical tasks.

Your dominant Dosha

What is my dominant dosha? Is there a way to determine my dosha type? With the advancement of the internet, people can now easily identity their dosha types by just browsing online, and answering a few questions. Not all of these online sources, though, are capable of delivering reliable and accurate results. Also, some of those sites may contain spam and malware. Fortunately, this book has a few links pertaining to the best and most trusted websites that provide free dosha quizzes. If you are interested in knowing your dosha type, make sure to check any of the links shared below.

http://www.yogajournal.com/health/2630

http://www.naturesformulary.com/contents/dosha-test

http://doshaquiz.chopra.com/

http://www.holisticonline.com/ayurveda/w_ayurveda-dtest1.htm

Your dosha makeup is a mere reflection of your ingrained tendencies, including your learning style, energy level, metabolism, temperament and a plethora of other aspects of your emotions, mind and body. Once you have identified your dosha, you may improve your general health by making the right choices to balance your body and mind.

3 THE BASICS OF BALANCING YOUR DOSHA FORCE

"Ayurveda is about nature; it's about seeing that we are connected to nature and that we have natural elements in ourselves. The less chemicals, preservatives, and artificial additives that you put on and inside your body, the healthier you're going to be and the less risk you have for getting sick. So, Ayurveda, in its essence, is about living purely and healthily and trying to achieve balance".

- Christy Turlington

Your dosha is a dynamic energy that changes frequently in response to your emotions, thoughts, actions, consumed foods and other neurological inputs that would feed your body and mind. When you live into the fulfillment of your individual nature, you naturally make dietary and lifestyle choices that create balance within your dosha. But when you start to live against your intrinsic nature, you will eventually be supporting unhealthy practices that can lead to mental and physical imbalances.

Vata

Are you a Vata type? Then, you should make sure to avoid stress at all cost. When you become too stressed, your Vata force becomes imbalanced, causing your activity begin to feel out of control. As a result, your mind endlessly races, which may lead to insomnia and anxiety. Additionally, you may begin to skip meals, resulting to digestion problems and unintended weight loss.

How Vata people become imbalanced

Going to sleep late in the evening

Following an unusual daily routine

Smoking cigarettes

Drinking black tea, coffee, or alcohol

Eating hastily

Eating while depressed or anxious

Eating foods that aggravate Vata

How to become balanced

Listen to calming and soothing music.

Get Ayurvedic massage on a regular basis.

Favor warm, heavy and sweet aromas like vanilla, sage, pine, lavender, frankincense, cloves, citrus, cinnamon, bay and basil.

Wear clothes that have warm and earth colors,

such as warm yellows, browns and pastels.

Make sure that your have regular bowel movements.

Light exercises that improve flexibility and balance are ideal for Vatta types.

Pitta

Pitta types, when in perfect balance, are intellectual beings with an exceptional ability to concentrate. As matter of fact, these people make good speakers, teachers and decision makers. But when they become overstressed and imbalanced, they become argumentative and short-tempered.

How Pitta people become imbalance

Being too competitive

Working too hard

Smoking cigarettes

Drinking black tea, coffee, or alcohol

Eating when angry or in foul mood

Eating foods that aggravate Pitta

How to become balanced

Balance activity and rest.

Indulge in an oil massage on a daily basis using

cool oils like olive and coconut.

Laugh as many times as you can every day.

Favor sweet and cooling aromas like chamomile, fennel, lavender, mint, jasmine, rose and sandalwood.

Kapha

The key to balancing your Kapha force is stimulation since this dosha type is inherently dense, heavy and cold. Kapha types, for the most part, cling to routine and status quo. Thus, as a Kapha type, you need a frequent stimulation of new experiences, sounds and sights.

How Kapha People become imbalance

Avoiding intellectual conversations and challenges

Spending most of their time indoors, specifically watching television on a couch

Lack of physical activity

Spending a lot of time in damp and climates

Eating to offset their emotions, such as indulging in sweet treats when not in the mood.

Overeating

Eating foods that aggravate Kapha

How to become balanced

Exercise every day to avoid accumulation and stagnation of toxins in your body.

Use stimulating and warm aromas like marjoram, juniper, eucalyptus, cinnamon, camphor, and cloves.

Favor bright and warm colors, such as red, orange and yellow.

Clean your space regularly to prevent clutter from accumulating in your physical offices, including your car, office and home.

Follow a solid daily routine. Ideally, you should wake on or before six o'clock in the morning. Also, don't take short naps during daytime.

4 THE AYURVEDA DIET

Unlike most diet fads, the Ayurvedic diet is more than just eating vegetables, fruits, rice and legumes. As a matter of fact, the basic principles of Ayurvedic diet can be applied to all sorts of cuisines, from Asian to Mediterranean. With the Ayurvedic diet, you get to consume a wide array of foods that help improve your overall well-being.

The philosophy of the diet

Food is truly an important aspect in every Ayurvedic practice. In Ayurveda, foods are downright essential for promoting happiness and general health. Foods, specifically the recommended ones, fortify the inner intelligence of your body, creating balance and harmony. This, in turn, helps prevents or cures an assortment of maladies and conditions.

"What we eat affects our emotions and can create a predisposition for both psychological and physical disorders. Just as wrong emotion can upset our digestion, so wrong digestion can upset our emotions."

-   Dr. David Frawley

The role of the six tastes

Ayurvedic practitioners believe that proper nutrition relies heavily on the tip of the tongue. As these practitioners have said, your sense of taste is your natural guide towards a healthy and balanced diet. For centuries, humans have used their taste buds to avoid toxicity as well as find healthy and nutritious foods. Not only does tour tongue determine tastes, but it can also unlock your food's nutritional value. Not to mention, they trigger the whole digestive process in your body.

In many ways, foods can speak to you directly through their tastes. For instance, a pulpy orange may reach out to you with a delightful message of pleasure. Likewise, a red-hot chili pepper may cry out to you in warning. As you tune into the various tastes that are naturally desired by your body, you are tapping information from your body's deep-seated wisdom pertaining to nutrition and food.

The six tastes and their roles

Ayurveda acknowledges the 6 tastes, and it is very important to include all these tastes in your daily diet. Each kind of taste feeds your spirit, senses, body and mind in its own peculiar way. Here are the 6 tastes and their roles to your health.

Sweet- Calms your nerves and builds tissues.

Sour – Improves mineral absorption as well as cleanses tissues.

Salty – Stimulates digestion, lubricates tissues, and adds more taste to your food.

Bitter – Lightens and detoxifies tissues.

Astringent- Dries fats, tightens tissues and absorbs water.

Pungent – Stimulates metabolism and digestion.

Common sources

Sweet – Milk, natural sugars, grains and fruits

Sour – Fermented foods, yogurt and sour fruits.

Salty – Sea vegetables and natural salts.

Bitter – Spices, herbs and dark leafy vegetables.

Astringent – Herbs, raw vegetables and fruits, as well as legumes.

The principles of Ayurvedic diet

With the 6 tastes, you get an easy-to-follow guide on how you can provide proper nourishment to your body. Instead of taking a look at the nutritional labels for protein and carbohydrate contents, your six tastes give you a better and more natural way of determining the nutritional needs of your body.

From a modern medical and nutritional perspective, your six tastes will gratify all the essential building blocks of your diet. For instance, sweet treats are practically high in water, carbohydrates, proteins and rich. Likewise, astringent and bitter foods are rich in minerals and vitamins.

Include all the six tastes in your meals

Your brain sends signals your body, when it needs food and energy. As you include all the six tastes into your meals, you are making sure that these signals are met adequately, preventing over-consumption of particular foods and food cravings.

Instilling the six tastes in every meal is not as complicated as a lot of people thought it would be. Honestly, it is a very simple a task that even kids can do. If, for instance, you need to satisfy your sour taste, you just have to add a squeeze of lemon to your cooked dish.

The six tastes can affect your dosha

Different food sources can cause particular doshas to either decrease or increase. For example, sweet foods help increase your Kapha, but it can decrease your Pitta and Vata doshas. With that said, you should consume the right proportions to your tastes based of your dominant dosha. You can do this by reading the next chapter.

5 BALANCE YOUR DOSHA WITH PROPER DIET

According to the philosophies of Ayurvedic medicine, aligning your diet to your dominant dosha is an absolute must, for optimal health. So, what are the foods best suited for my dosha makeup? And, how do I balance the six tastes according to my dominant dosha? To answer these questions, continue reading the pointers shared in this chapter.

As an Ayurvedic follower or practitioner, you must indulge in foods that will have a balancing effect on your dominant dosha. Also, if your dosha has become aggravated or excessive, try to eat foods that will help stabilize (pacify) it.

"Let food be thy medicine, thy medicine shall be thy food."

Hippocrates

The recommended Vata diet

Is Vata your dominant dosha? Since your dosha type is light, cooling and drying, consume foods that are heavy, warming and oily. As for the tastes, the best ones that pacify this dosha are sour, salty and sweet. You should try to cut down on foods that astringent, bitter and pungent.

Ideal Vata foods:

Grains – Wheat products, basmati rice and cooked oatmeal

Legumes – Whole mung beans, red lentils and yellow split mung beans

Vegetables – Zucchini, tomato, potato, sweet potato, winter squash, yellow squash, spinach, radish, white pumpkin, okra, tender eggplant, cucumber, celery root, carrot, bok choy, beets, and artichoke

Spices – Sea salt, tamarind, mustard seeds, hing, ginger, fried garlic, fenugreek, fennel, cumin, coriander, clove, cinnamon, cardamom, black pepper and anise.

Seeds and nuts

Oils

Sweeteners – Honey, fructose, date sugar and sugar cane products

Dairy – Sour cream, panir, non-aged soft cheeses, yogurt, milk, ghee, cream and butter

Fruits: All sweet and ripe juicy fruits like

avocado, banana, cherries and apricots

Meat: White meats are good, but only in small amounts.

Foods to reduce

Grains – Rye, row oats, millet, corn, and barley

Legumes – All except for red lentils and yellow mung beans

Vegetables – Raw vegetables, orange squash, sprouts, potato, green leafy vegetables, celery stalk, mature eggplant and broccoli cauliflower

Spices – Raw garlic, chili peppers, cayenne and other forms of hot spices

Sweeteners – Artificial sweeteners

Dairy – Powdered dairy products, hard cheese and ice-cream

Fruits – Unripe fruits like persimmon, guava and cranberries

Meat- Red meat

The recommended Pitta diet

For Pitta types, favoring liquids and cool foods is vital, since an excess of this dosha overheats the body and mind. The best tastes for this dosha are astringent, bitter and sweet. Foods that are sour, salty and pungent must be reduced.

Ideal Pitta foods:

Grains – Couscous, amaranth, kamut, quinoa, oats, barley and white rice

Legumes – Soy bean products (non-fermented), small kidney beans and mung beans

Vegetables – Green leafy vegetables (except spinach), sweet corn, winter squash, bok choy, kale, cucumber, chard, lettuce, sprouts, sweet potato, celery, green beans, cabbage, broccoli, yellow squash, artichokes, and asparagus

Dairy – Panir, cream cheese, cream, sweet lassi and milk

Sweeteners – Date sugar, and whole natural sugar cane

Oils – Sunflower, olive and ghee

Seeds and nuts – Blanched almonds (small quantities), as well as pumpkin and sunflower seeds

Spices – Marjoram, oregano, basil, thyme, black pepper, cinnamon, ginger root, cardamom, saffron, turmeric, cumin, and coriander

Fruits – Banana, raisins, papaya, plums, sweet pineapple, sweet oranges, kiwi, melons, avocado and sweet grapes

Foods to reduce

General – Acidic foods and beverages, vinegar, and hot and spicy foods

Grains – Brown rice, buckwheat, rye, millet and corn

Vegetables – Seaweed, spinach, beets, carrots, onions, radish and tomato

Fruits – Cherries, lime, lemon, prunes, berries, sour pineapple sour grapes, peaches and grapefruit

Sweeteners – Honey, brown sugar and molasses

Nuts

Oils – Canola, sesame, safflower, corn and almond

Spices – Asafetida, mustard, catsup, fenugreek, celery seeds, cloves, mustard seeds, garlic, onion and chili peppers

The recommended Kapha diet

Warm, dry and light foods are ideal for Kapha types, as this dosha type is cold, oily and heavy by nature. What are the preferred tastes for this dosha? As a Kapha person, you should favor Kapha-pacifying foods with astringent, bitter and pungent tastes. Likewise, try to reduce eating foods with salty, sour and sweet tastes.

Ideal Kapha foods

Grains – Wheat, oats, rice, rye, buckwheat, corn, millet, barley, and old grains (one year)

Legumes – All are acceptable except for tofu

Vegetables – Tender radish, tender eggplant, tomato, green papaya, okra, zucchini, white pumpkin, sprouts, pepper, peas, broccoli, cauliflower, beet root, cabbage, carrot, and green leafy vegetables

Dairy – Whole milk, ghee (small amounts), low-fat milk, as well as butter and lassi milk

Sweeteners – Honey

Oils – Sesame, corn and mustard

Seeds and nuts – Pumpkin and sunflower

Spices –All spices except for salt

Fruits – Guava, papaya, apple, peaches, dates, digs, raisins, cranberries, persimmon, grapes, jambu, cashew and pomegranate

Foods to reduce

General – Avoid eating large servings of food, especially in the evening

Grains – New grains like rice and wheat

Legumes – Tofu or soy beans

Vegetables- tapioca and sweet potatoes

Dairy – Butter, cream and yoghurt

Nuts

Fruits – Apricot, coconut, mango, plums, melons, oranges, pineapple, banana, and avocado

Spices – Slat

Meat – Red meat

6 A COMPELLING EXERCISE ROUTINE FOR YOUR DOSHA

"Life is one percent what happens to you, and ninety-nine percent how you respond to it."

- Shubhra Krishan, Essential Ayurveda: What It Is and What It Can Do For You

Exercise is, without a doubt, very essential in any Ayurvedic practice. With exercise, Ayurvedic practitioners become firmer as well a more tolerant to hardships. What's more, it stimulates digestion, eliminates impurities, relives stress and reverses the process of aging. As the studies of Drs. Irwin Rosenberg and William Evans from Tufts University have confirmed, exercise enhances the key aging biomarkers, such as aerobic capacity, strength, bone density, and muscle mass.

Do you want to keep your body in good condition for a long time? Then, you need to exercise on a regular basis. This, however, does not mean beating yourself up with heavy dumbbells and endless sets of push-ups. From an Ayurvedic perspective, exercise is designed to make you feel happy, refreshed, and ready for the remaining activities of the day. In Ayurveda, you don't have to pound yourself to exhaustion, and take painkillers to manage the pain from your vigorous workouts.

Today, a lot of people struggle in keeping up with an exercise program. For the most part, these people consider exercise as a boring and tedious chore that they have to do daily. Luckily, there is a way to make exercise more intriguing and exciting. The secret to making exercise a fun endeavor is to know your dosha type, and find out the physical activities that align perfectly with your dosha vibe.

Kapha Types

Blessed with amazing physical strength and steady energy, Kapha types will normally excel at sports that require great feats of strength and endurance, such as rowing, dancing, aerobics, and even contact sports like rugby and soccer. Yet, for all their physical gifts, Kapas may sometimes lack the motivation they need to work out. Moreover, they can often feel sluggish and sapped of energy, especially when they haven't been exercising for a long time.

Are you a Kapha who is feeling a bit sluggish lately? To clear sluggishness and congestion in your Kapha force, you may do any type of aerobic activity, as long as it gives you a good sweat. Also, you may break your laziness by taking a short walk or jog (around 30 minutes or less).

Do you want to have significant improvements in

your vitality? As you exercise, wear a two-layer outfit, and do your best to experience heavy sweating. Progressively, move to the more challenging exercises like cycling and hiking.

Pitta Types

Thanks to their strong will and drive, Pitta people tend to take on the more advanced and challenging sports, such as mountain climbing, tennis, hiking and skiing. But since Pittas are naturally competitive, they have to be a tad more cautious not to increase their levels of stress when exercising. As athletes, Pittas normally stew over every bad shot, and are the ones who want to win the game at all costs.

Is Pitta dominating your body's force? If so, you are most likely fond of winter sports, as Pittas can handle colder temperatures a lot better than their counterparts. While Pitta types don't have the uncanny endurance of Kaphas, they perform quite well in any exercise, provided that it is done in moderation.

As a Kapha, you might want to try rollerblading and long-distance bicycling. In addition, taking a walk in a scenic outdoor are can be very beneficial to you. As you take a leisurely walk, you'll get to replenish your senses and enjoy a taste of nature's majestic beauty and tranquil charm.

Last, but not the least, swimming is a fun and breathtaking exercise that Pittas would surely love.

With swimming, Pittas get submerge in relaxing waters that cool down the heat of their dominant dosha, reliving their body from the tension accumulated throughout the day.

Vata Types

Vatas are, by nature, enthusiastic, and have bursts of energy within their body. Sadly, they are more likely to get tired quickly than the Kaphas and Pittas. Also, when Vata people become imbalanced, they tend to get carried away and push themselves too hard.

A person, with a dominant Vata force, greatly benefits from taking up ground exercises like dancing, bicycling, walking and easy. When done in moderation, these exercises can develop his or her agility, balance and strength. During the winter season, indoor sports are optimal for Vata people since they are inept in cold climates. Plus, they don't have enough muscles and fats to protect themselves from the colder elements.

Choosing the right exercise type of exercise offers a plethora of benefits to your mind, body and spirit. Besides, it makes your routine more exciting, and can provide you a sense of fulfillment. But if you are following a program for the sake of maintaining your health, without enjoying it a bit, you are likely to end it prematurely. So, create an exciting exercise routine that is perfectly suited for your body-mind type with the hints shared above.

7 HOW TO INCORPORATE AYURVEDA IN YOUR LIFE

Have you ever wondered how you can incorporate the Ayurvedic principles into your modern and bustling lifestyle? A lot of people nowadays have considered making this kind of lifestyle change, but most of them assume that they don't have time to incorporate its principles into their lifestyle. Little do they know, instilling Ayurveda doesn't need a great deal of time to make its magic work into their frantic life.

While the world has progressed significantly from the Stone Age to the Digital Age, people unfortunately have regressed from their roots, and have lived in a rather superficial fashion. They have become less conscious of their well-being and health, and are constantly bombarded with buzzing noise, leading to anxiety, stress as well as poor physical and mental health. But with Ayurveda, you get to learn compelling ancient principles that will your spirit, body, soul and mind. Best of all, these principles help boost your overall health.

"Because we cannot scrub our inner body, we need

to learn a few skills to help cleanse our tissues, organs, and mind. This is the art of Ayurveda."

- Sebastian Pole, Discovering the True You with Ayurveda

Vata

Is Vata is your dominant dosha? To incorporate Ayurveda into your life, try going to bed before 10 in the evening, and wake up at 6 in the morning. As much as possible, avoid watching television or using the computer late at night. That way, you are instilling the ancient principles of Ayurveda as well as add more balance to your Vata dosha. More importantly, it makes you feel fresher and more energized.

As a Vata type, one of the best ways you can incorporate Ayurveda into your life is to experience a reinvigorating Ayurvedic massage treatment from a trained therapist. In many ways, a massage treatment opens the doors to the world Ayurveda. In addition, it helps create balance to your Vata vibe, helping you practice the principles of this ancient art.

Pitta

Spend some time with Mother Nature by trekking in the woods, walking in the moonlight, or keeping fresh flowers and plants in your office and home. Basically, nature helps unlock your true potential, as a Pitta person. Also, it replenishes your energy, and provides emotional, mental and physical peace without straining your body.

Don't have the time to do it? No matter how busy you are, you must make it a point to get in touch in nature. Besides, there are a lot of city parks and gardens that can somehow give you a slice of nature's offerings.

Kapha

Kapha types tend to be overindulgent and sluggish. As a result, they can become a little overweight, and would hold on to their inner energy. Are you a Kapha person? To incorporate the practices of Ayurveda into your life, first you need to clean up your space. Then, get regular exercise, to get rid of the toxins and sluggishness in your body.

Of course, to fully incorporate the principles of this ancient Indian art, you need to eat the foods that provide balance to your body-mind type. Likewise, don't forget to exercise regularly with the physical activities best suited to your dominant force. Once you are able to do all these things, your life will become more balanced and harmonious.

8 CONCLUSION

Ayurveda is an efficacious and reliable form of alternative medicine that has been embraced by millions of people from all over the world. As a matter of fact, a lot of world-famous media figures have gone holistic with Ayurvedic medicine, including Deepak Chopra, Dr. Oz, Oprah and Christy Turlington. An ancient Indian holistic approach, Ayurveda can greatly benefit your mind, body and spirit in a multitude of ways.

Ayurveda is, in essence, a way of life that gives you emotional and spiritual peace. While most people consider it as a treatment for certain disorders, Ayurveda can be a path to balance within the body and ultimate happiness in life. And why not? With Ayurveda, you get to naturally transform yourself into a better, healthier and happier person and what could be more valuable than that?

9 BONUS RECIPES

Frying Spices

Description: Frying spice brings out the flavor and health benefits of essential oils.

Ingredients:

ghee

mustard seeds

cumin

other spices (depending on dosha)

ginger

coriander

turmeric

Directions:

1. Heat ghee in skillet over medium high heat.

2. Add a few mustard seeds, when the seeds start to pop turn the heat to medium.
3. Add the rest of seeds and as they pop add cumin seeds then add other seeds and spices.
4. When popping slows add ginger and sauté until golden brown.
5. Add coriander seeds for 20 seconds and then turmeric for 10 seconds
6. Now you're ready to use this spice for tomatoes or other vegetables for curry.

Ghee

Description: This is a simple recipe for Ghee, which is clarified butter.

Ingredients:

One or more pounds of unsalted butter

Directions:

1. Place butter in a heavy medium-size saucepan.
2. Simmer over medium heat while stirring. Be careful not to burn.
3. The milk solids will separate and settle in the bottom of the pan.
4. After about 15 min. remove from heat and pass through a sieve.
5. Place in a sterile sealed jar.

6. There is no need to refrigerate ghee. Store for up to 3 months in a cool, dark place.

Ginger Tea

Description:

A refreshing beverage that is popular in Ayurvedic treatment for eliminating toxins and ama if taken regularly. You may use fresh gingerroot (adrak) or dried ginger (saunth).

Ingredients:

One or more cups of water

2 or 3 Slices of ginger

1 teaspoon. Of lemon juice (optional)

1 teaspoon. Of honey (optional)

Directions:

1. Place water in pot with ginger slices and bring to a boil.
2. It will start to fizz, turn down heat.
3. Simmer for about 5 minutes. until dark yellow.
4. Add optional ingredients if you like

Mango Chutney

Description: Use as a condiment with any meal. Be sure to choose hard mangoes for this recipe.

Ingredients:

2 large green slightly under-ripe mangoes

2 cups sugar

6 tablespoon white vinegar

1½ teaspoon salt

1 teaspoon fenugreek seeds

1 small cinnamon stick

5 black cardamom pods (opened to expose seeds)

½ teaspoon nigella seeds

20 cloves

1 teaspoon black peppercorns

Directions:

1. Peel mangoes and julienne 1 – 1½ pieces.
2. Discard seed and place into large pot.
3. Stir in all spices.
4. Bring to boil stirring 4 – 5 minutes, reduce heat.
5. Cover the pan and simmer until slightly thick about 15 minutes (chutney will thicken while it cools also).
6. Let chutney cool completely and place in sterile fruit jar.
7. Keeps the same as preserves.

Bonus Recipes: Savory
Chickpea Flour Pancakes

Description: (Cheela ka besan) This Indian crêpe-like "pancake" can be used to roll up leftover vegetable curry for a satisfying lunch.

Ingredients:

½ cup besan (chickpea flour)

3 tablespoon chapati flour (or substitute all-purpose wheat flour)

 pinch turmeric powder

½ teaspoon minced ginger (or a pinch of ginger powder if fresh ginger is unavailable)

⅓ teaspoon cumin powder

¼ teaspoon paprika

¼ teaspoon salt

1 to 1½ cup water

1 tablespoon sesame seeds

a few pieces minced cilantro

ghee or oil for cooking

Directions:

- Mix dry ingredients with a whisk to remove lumps.
- Add enough water to make a medium-thick batter (not stiff, not runny). The amount of water that you will need depends on the flours that you are using.
- Add all remaining ingredients except ghee or oil and mix well.
- Let stand for about 15 minutes.
- Heat a small amount of ghee or oil in a nonstick crepe pan (or a pan with low sides).
- When the pan is hot, pour in about ⅓ cup of batter. Rotate the pan so that the batter spreads out.
- Cook for a few minutes before turning the pancake to cook on the other side.
- Keep warm in oven until you have used up all the batter.

Curried Vegetables with Mango Chutney

Description: Serve this dish with basmati rice and Mango Chutney

Ingredients:

2 tablespoon ghee

¼ tablespoon grated ginger

1 teaspoon fennel

¼ teaspoon turmeric

1 onion chopped

¼ teaspoon sea salt

¼ cup peas

2 cups cabbage (substitutions/additions- broccoli, squash, carrot)

2 tablespoon besan flour (chickpea flour)

1 blanched tomato

4 tablespoon water

2 tablespoon yogurt

Cilantro (optional)

Directions:

1. In a large saucepan over medium heat, heat ghee add onion sauté, when onion is lightly golden add other spices continue to sauté.
2. While sautéing, in separate pot steam vegetables.
3. Add besan flour to curry and cook 5 minutes.
4. Then add water, then yogurt, and vegetables.
5. Garnish with cilantro and serve with mango chutney on side.

Mung Dahl

Description: Ayurvedic healers recommend the mung bean and its split version, mung dal for all body-types because it's nutritious and easy to digest.

Ingredients:

1 cup of dried mung dahl (lentils)

2 tablespoon brown mustard seeds

1 medium size Onion (chopped)

7 cloves of garlic (finely chopped)

1" ginger root (grated or finely chopped)

1 teaspoon turmeric

3 green or black cardamom pods (cracked)

2 small red chilies (or ¼ t. Cayenne)

3 cloves

3 bay leaves or a pinch of neem leaves

½ teaspoon coriander seeds

¼ teaspoon cinnamon

1 pinch saffron

¼ teaspoon black salt

2 tablespoon ghee

Directions:

1. Melt the ghee in a large pot.
2. Add the mustard seeds, cover the pot, and wait for the seeds to pop. Add the seeds, sauté lightly.
3. Dice the onion and sauté until translucent. Add the garlic and ginger, sauté a little longer.
4. Add the rice and lentils and cover with water twice the depth of the rice and lentils.
5. Bring to a boil, and then reduce the heat.
6. Add the powdered spices (turmeric, cayenne) and the coriander, cinnamon, bay or neem leaves, saffron, cloves, and cardamom.
7. When the lentils are tender, add the salt.
8. For extra energy, use a few pieces of astragalus or kombu.

Spicy Rice Paneer

Ingredients:

1/4 Paneer cubed

1/2 cup basmati rice

2 tbs. Raisins

1/2 teaspoon whole coriander seeds

1 tbs. fresh grated ginger

1/4 red bell pepper (optional)

1 tbs. cilantro

1 teaspoon coarsely ground black pepper

1/4 teaspoon salt

Directions:

1. Rinse rice three or more times until water is almost clear.
2. Boil water, add rice and salt.
3. Simmer for 15-20 minutes.
4. Remove from heat let stand for 5 minutes to firm.
5. Sauté ginger until golden
6. Add coriander and bell pepper
7. Place in dish fluff rice and add remaining ingredients.

Garnish with cilantro and serve.

Bonus Recipes: Sweet

Cherry Tea Biscuits

Description: These nearly fatless biscotti-style cookies are idea for dipping.

Ingredients:

1 cup chopped cherries

1 cup pistachios

⅓ cup rum

4 egg whites and 2 eggs

2 teaspoon vanilla extract

1 teaspoon almond extract

1 tablespoon orange zest

⅔ cups sugar

1¾ plain flour

1 cup whole wheat flour

2 teaspoon cinnamon

2 teaspoon baking powder

1 cup unprocessed wheat bran

Directions:

1. In a saucepan simmer cherries and rum over medium heat.
2. Preheat oven to 350°F.
3. Stir and cover to let set for 10 minutes, uncover and cool for 10 minutes.
4. Cover a baking sheet with foil and coat with non-stick cooking spray.
5. Sift all-purpose flour, whole wheat flour, baking powder, sugar, and cinnamon.
6. Stir in wheat bran.
7. In a mixing bowl, whisk egg whites, egg, orange zest, vanilla and almond extracts until smooth.
8. Whisk in cherry and rum mixture.
9. Stir in dry ingredients until well combined.
10. Turn dough onto floured work surface and divide in half.
11. Flour each half and shape to a log.
12. Place logs onto baking sheet and bake until light brown and puffed approx. 20 minutes.
13. Cool 10 min. or up to several hours.
14. Transfer logs to work surface and cut into biscotti-style pieces.
15. Put back in oven for 12 minutes. turn and brown on both sides 6 minutes. each.
16. Let cool and store in container or serve warm.

Cinnamon-baked Pears

Description: When you think dessert start with

something that is nutritious then add spices for flavor.

Ingredients:

1 stick cinnamon

¼ cup dates, chopped

¼ cup raisins

½ teaspoon cinnamon or 1 cinnamon stick

1 teaspoon lemon zest

2 tablespoon prune purée

2 tablespoon brown sugar

4 large pears

½ cup water

Directions:

1. In a mixing bowl, mash first 7 ingredients until you have a paste.
2. Keeping the stem intact, peel/core pears, digging out a cavity 1 in. across and 2½ in. deep from the center of the large end.
3. Press equal parts mixture into pears.
4. Place pears standing up in a small baking dish, add water and cinnamon stick to pan, cover with foil.

5. In a 325°F preheated oven, bake pears 40 minutes or until tender.
6. Transfer pears to individual plates and pour remaining syrup from baking pan on top.
7. Place a dollop of yogurt cheese next to each pear and serve.

Mango Lassi

Description: This drink dates back to ancient times. It's a nice drink for the summer months that aids in digestion. Ayurveda recommends yogurt to be taken in this form if you are trying to lose weight. Enjoy it with a spicy Indian meal or alone.

Ingredients Edit

2 cups plain yogurt

2 cups water

½ cup sugar or honey

2 – 3 ripe mangoes or 1 can mango pulp.

Directions:

1. Process all ingredients in a blender.
2. Enjoy!

Stewed Apple and Clove

Description: Perfect Ayurvedic breakfast, lunch, or snack for increased vitality.

Ingredients:

1 Apple cored and peeled

5 whole cloves

1/4 cup water

Directions:

1. Dice Apple
2. Add cloves and water
3. Cook Apples until soft
4. Discard clove cool slightly and serve

Sunshine Balls

Ingredients:

1/2 cup plus 2 tablespoons toasted sunflower seeds

1/2 cup shredded, unsweetened coconut (omit for Kapha)

2-3 tablespoons Raisins (omit for Vata)

1/4 cup sunflower butter

1 tablespoon maple syrup

1 teaspoon almond extract

1/2 teaspoon coriander powder

Directions:

1. Grind the sunflower seeds in a blender to a coarse meal.
2. Mix all the ingredients together in a mixing bowl and press into1 inch balls.

Recipes references: Recipes Wikia.

MORE FROM THIS AUTHOR

Below you'll find some of my other books that are popular on Amazon and Kindle as well.

No Drugs, No Lenses. How to Improve Vision Naturally: Effective Exercises and Techniques to Improve Your Eyesight Naturally

Natural Health Vitamin Recipes: How to Make Delicious Natural Vitamins & Nourishing Vitamin Water at Home

10745883R00035

Printed in Great Britain
by Amazon.co.uk, Ltd.,
Marston Gate.